What Happens Next? Dealing with Life Changes

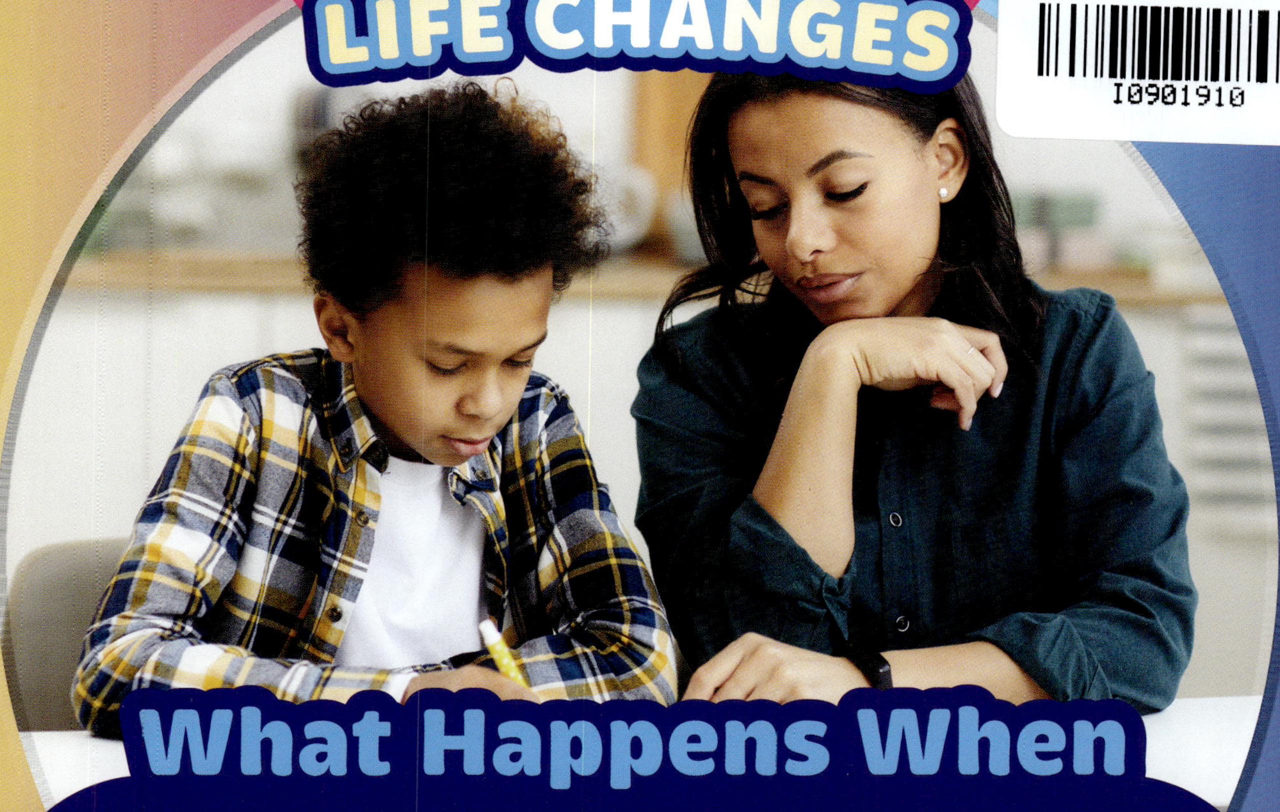

What Happens When I Have a Learning Difference?

Janey Levy

PowerKiDS press.

Published in 2025 by The Rosen Publishing Group, Inc.
2544 Clinton Street, Buffalo, NY 14224

First Edition

Editor: Theresa Emminizer
Book Design: Leslie Taylor

Photo Credits: Cover SeventyFour/Shutterstock.com; p. 5 (top) Pra Chid/Shutterstock.com, PeopleImages.com - Yuri A (bottom) /Shutterstock.com; p. 7 (top) Loredana Sangiuliano/Shutterstock.com, (bottom) Denis Makarenko/Shutterstock.com; p. 9 (Cher) Tom Rose/Shutterstock.com, (inset) LEE SNIDER PHOTO IMAGES/Shutterstock.com; p. 11 (books) SJBright/Shutterstock.com, (inset) spatuletail/Shutterstock.com; p. 13 Featureflash Photo Agency/Shutterstock.com; p. 15 (Simone) Fetr Toman/Shutterstock.com, (Greta) DFree/Shutterstock.com; p. 17 Studio Romantic/Shutterstock.com; p. 19 Kathy Hutchins/Shutterstock.com; p. 21 Ground Picture/Shutterstock.com.

Cataloging-in-Publication Data

Names: Levy, Janey.
Title: What happens when I have a learning difference? / Janey Levy.
Description: Buffalo, NY : PowerKids Press, 2025. | Series: What happens next? dealing with life changes| Includes glossary and index.
Identifiers: ISBN 9781725327092 (pbk.) | ISBN 9781725327115 (library bound) | ISBN 9781725327122 (ebook)
Subjects: LCSH: Learning disabilities--Juvenile literature. | Dyslexia--Juvenile literature. | Attention-deficit hyperactivity disorder--Juvenile literature.
Classification: LCC LC4704.74 L48 2025 | DDC 371.9--dc23

Manufactured in the United States of America

Some of the images in this book illustrate individuals who are models. The depictions do not imply actual situations or events.

CPSIA Compliance Information: Batch #CSPK25. For Further Information contact Rosen Publishing at 1-800-237-9932.

CONTENTS

Learning Differently 4
Rough Times with Reading 6
Math Misery 8
Wrestling with Writing 10
Moving Your Body 12
ADHD 14
School Plans 16
You Can Do It! 18
Talk About It 20
Glossary 22
For More Information 23
Index 24

Learning Differently

Learning is a doorway to all kinds of worlds. You can discover the past and the present; animals and plants; Earth, the sun, and the moon. But not everyone learns the same way.

Some people learn best with pictures. Some learn best by listening. Some learn best by doing. However, other learning differences can make certain tasks harder. These come from differences in the brain and how the brain **processes** information, or facts and knowledge. Let's learn more about some of these!

Your Point of View

It's important to remember that a learning difference doesn't have anything to do with how smart you are. Lots of very smart people have learning differences.

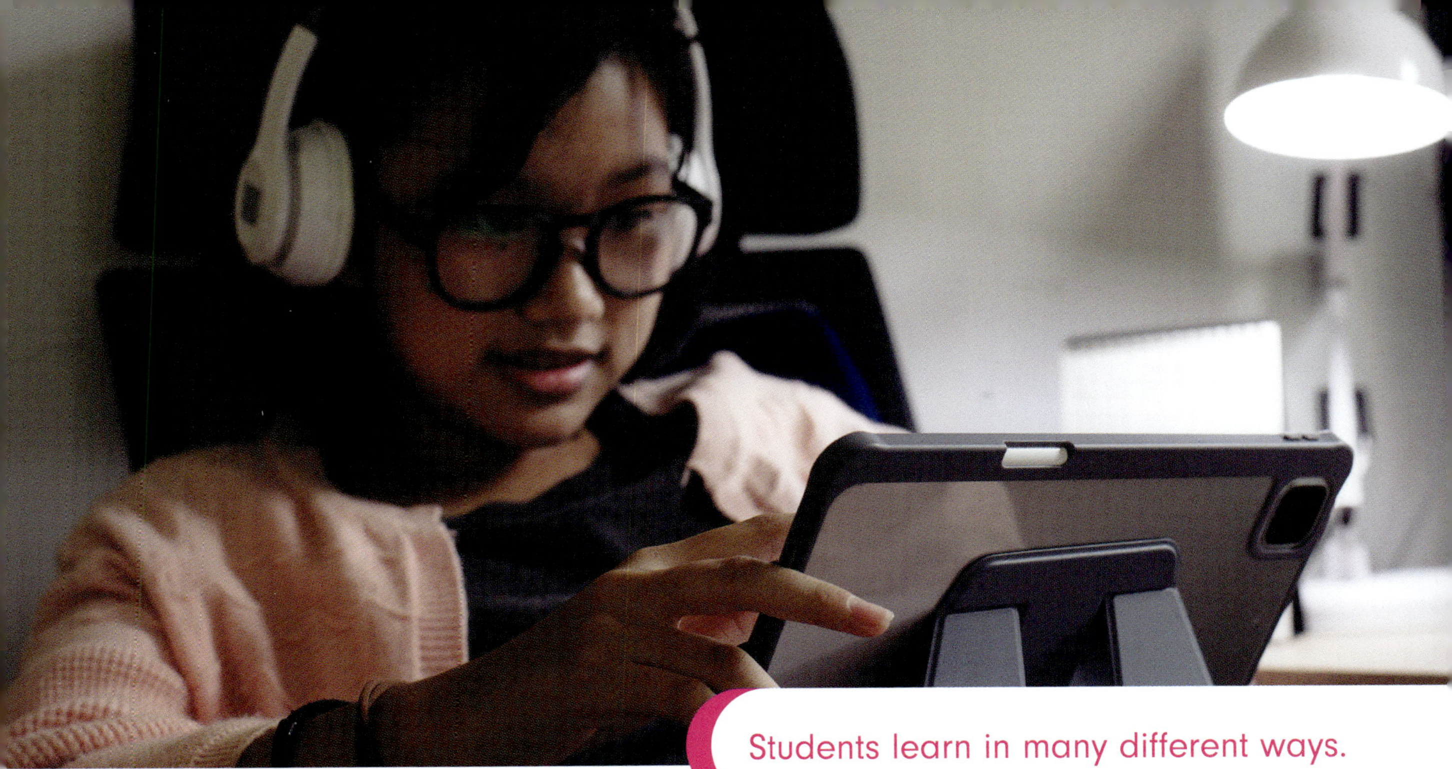

Students learn in many different ways.

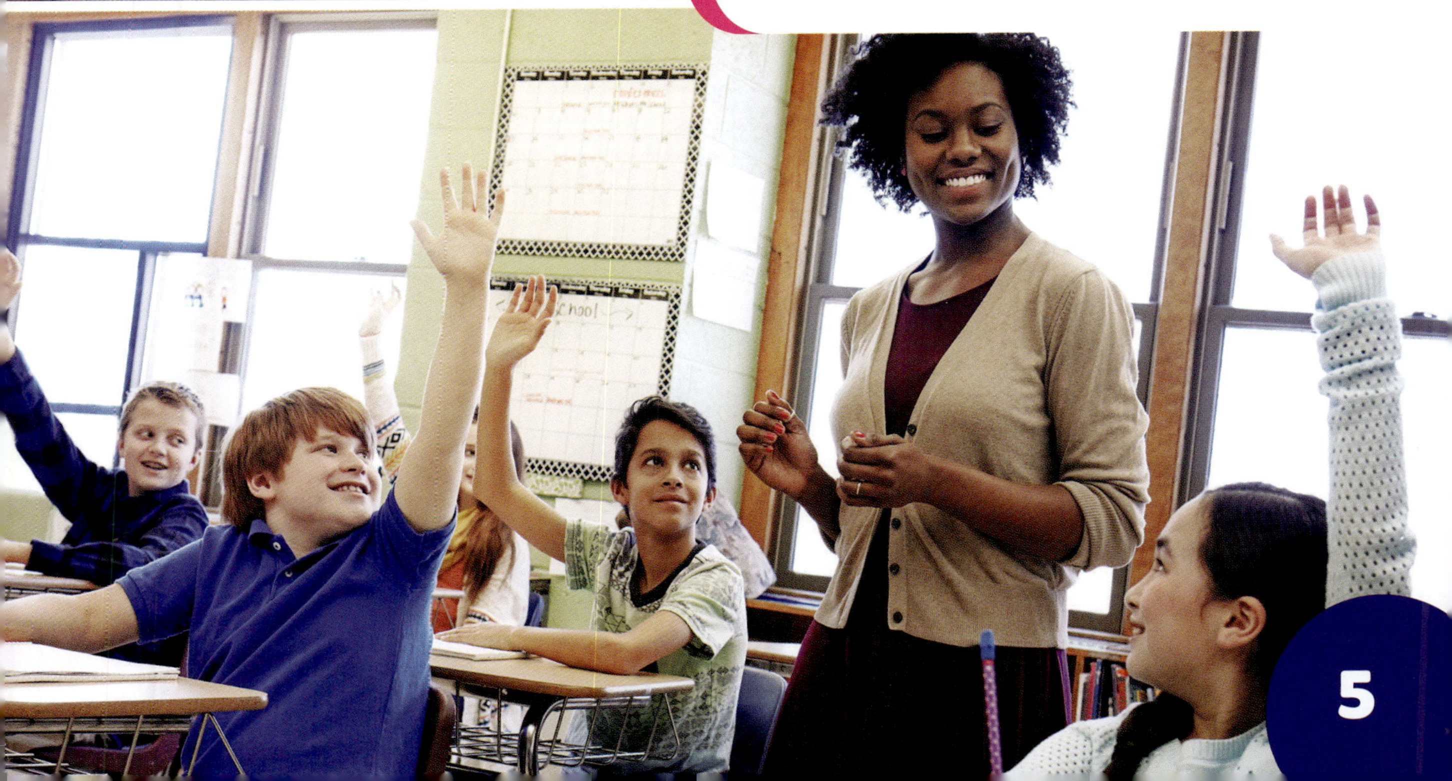

Rough Times with Reading

The most common learning difference affects, or acts on, a person's reading skills. In fact, it affects all language skills. It's called dyslexia (dihs-LEHK-see-uh).

With dyslexia, your brain sees and hears words differently. Letters may jump around or mix together. Sounds in words may change around. Words that sound alike may get mixed up. Letters that look alike—such as *d* and *b* or *p* and *q*—may get mixed up. These brain differences can make reading, spelling, and sometimes talking hard.

Your Point of View

Did you know that George Washington, the first U.S. president, couldn't spell correctly? It's believed he had dyslexia!

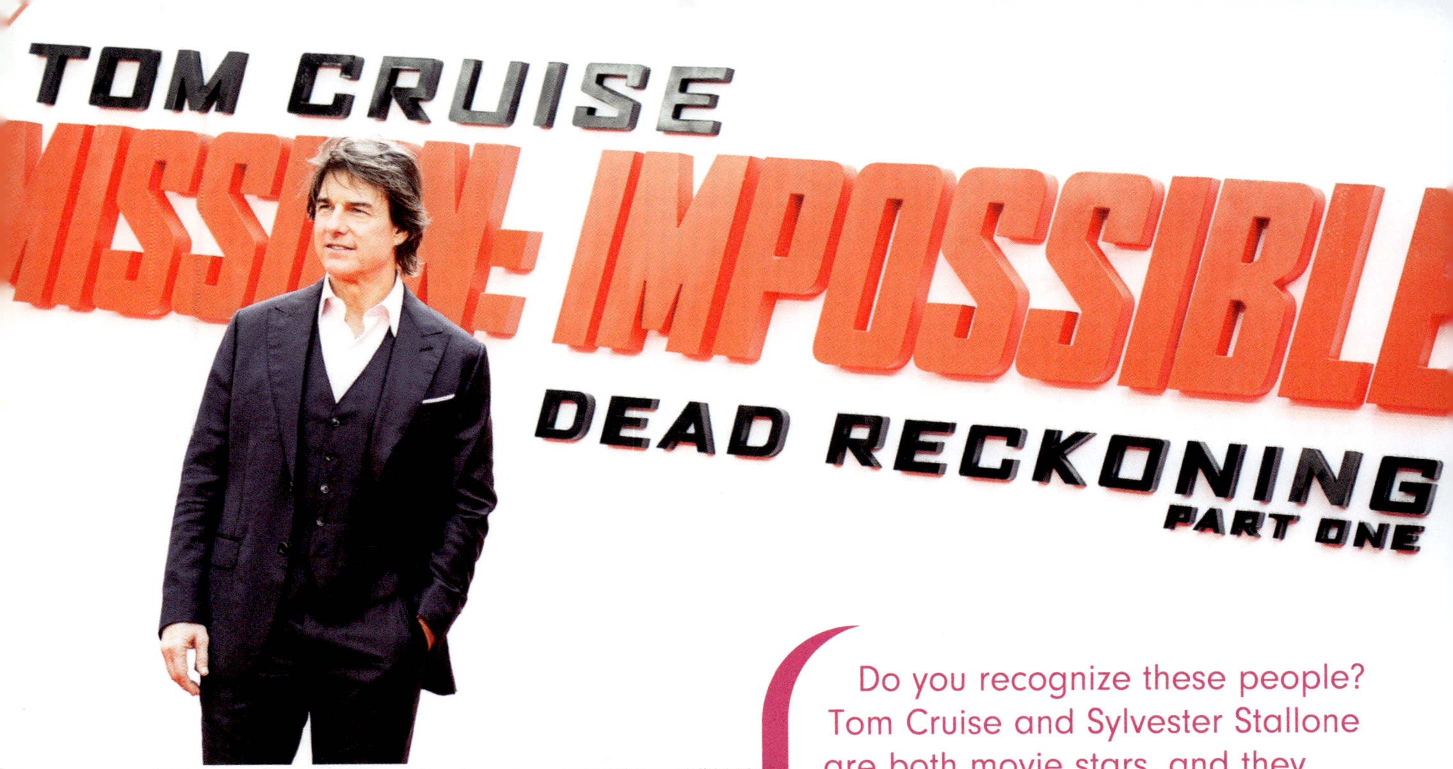

Do you recognize these people? Tom Cruise and Sylvester Stallone are both movie stars, and they both have dyslexia. Stallone writes movies too!

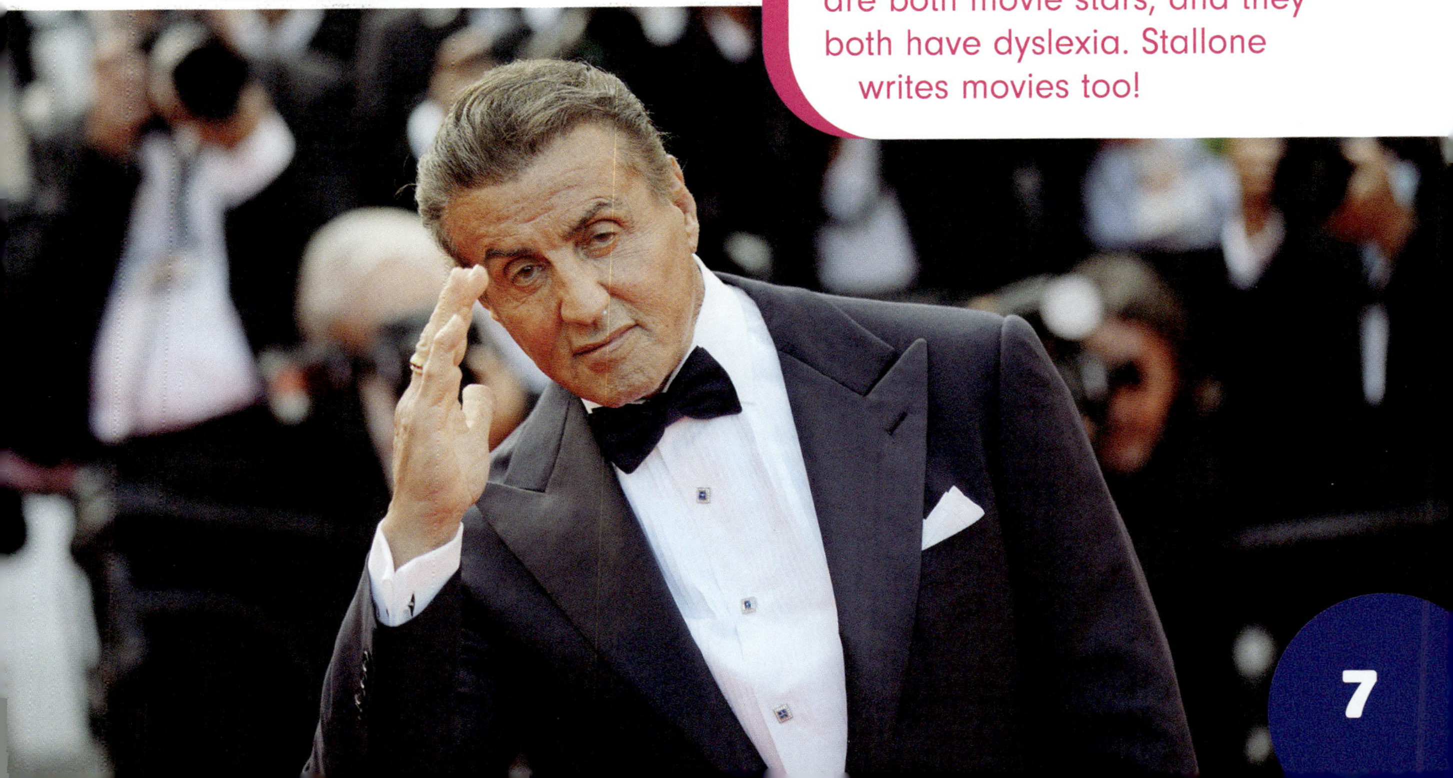

Math Misery

Another learning difference affects your ability to do math or anything having to do with numbers. It's called dyscalculia (dihs-kaal-KYU-lee-uh).

With dyscalculia, your brain has trouble with simple math operations like adding and subtracting. Math signs like + and – may get mixed up. Telling time and remembering numbers such as phone numbers may be hard. It may be hard to connect a written number, such as 7, with its matching word, *seven*. Telling left from right also may be hard!

Your Point of View

Benjamin Franklin was one of the **Founding Fathers** of the United States and was also famous for his many science experiments and inventions. It's believed he had dyscalculia!

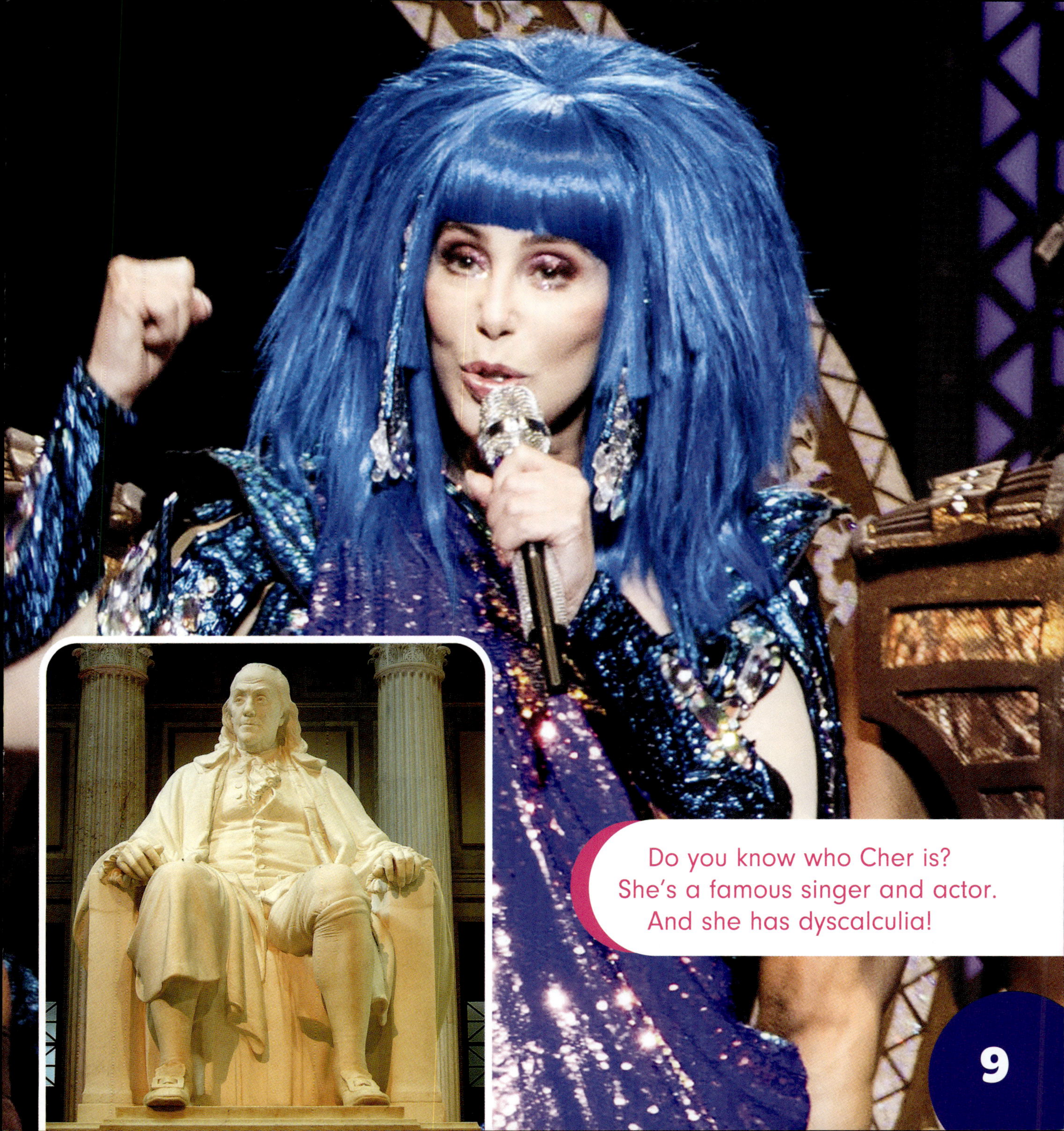

Do you know who Cher is? She's a famous singer and actor. And she has dyscalculia!

Wrestling with Writing

Another common learning difference causes problems with writing. It's called dysgraphia (dihs-GRA-fee-uh).

If you have dysgraphia, your writing may be messy. You may write letters backward. You may have problems with letter size and spacing between letters. You may write slowly and have problems writing in a straight line. Spelling may be hard for you. You may leave out words in sentences or put the words in the wrong order. You may also have trouble holding and controlling a pencil or pen.

Your Point of View

Have you heard of Louis Pasteur? This famous scientist invented pasteurization, the process of heating milk to kill bacteria and make it safe to drink. And he had dysgraphia!

This is Agatha Christie, who may have had dysgraphia. But problems with writing didn't keep her from becoming one of the most famous mystery writers of the 20th century! Many movies have been made based on her books. And people are still turning her books into movies!

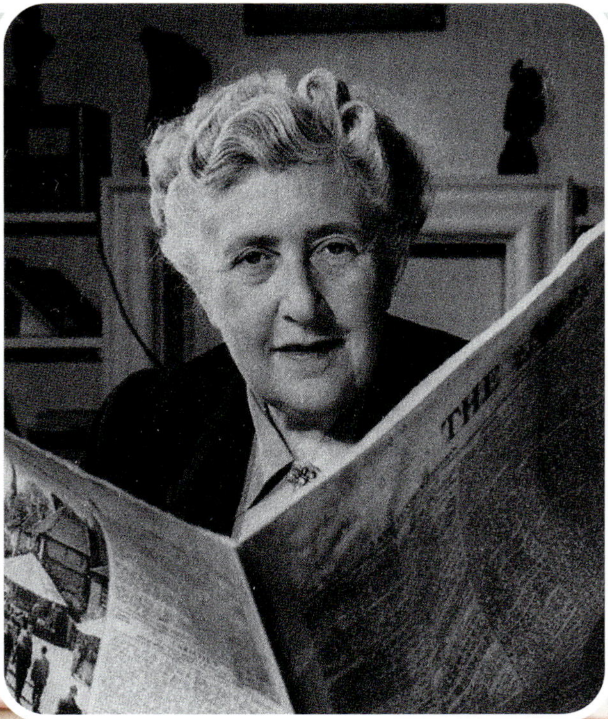

Moving Your Body

Another learning difference affects **coordination** and the ability to get your **muscles** to work properly to carry out movements. It's called dyspraxia (dihs-PRAK-see-uh).

With dyspraxia, you may fall and bump into things a lot. Going up and down stairs may be hard. Activities such as riding a bike, jumping, and playing sports may be hard. You may have trouble writing, drawing, and using **scissors**. You may have trouble doing buttons, tying your shoes, brushing your teeth, and even talking clearly.

Your Point of View

Emma Lewell-Buck has dyspraxia. You might not have heard of her, but she's a member of Parliament, the British lawmaking body. Her dyspraxia hasn't stopped her!

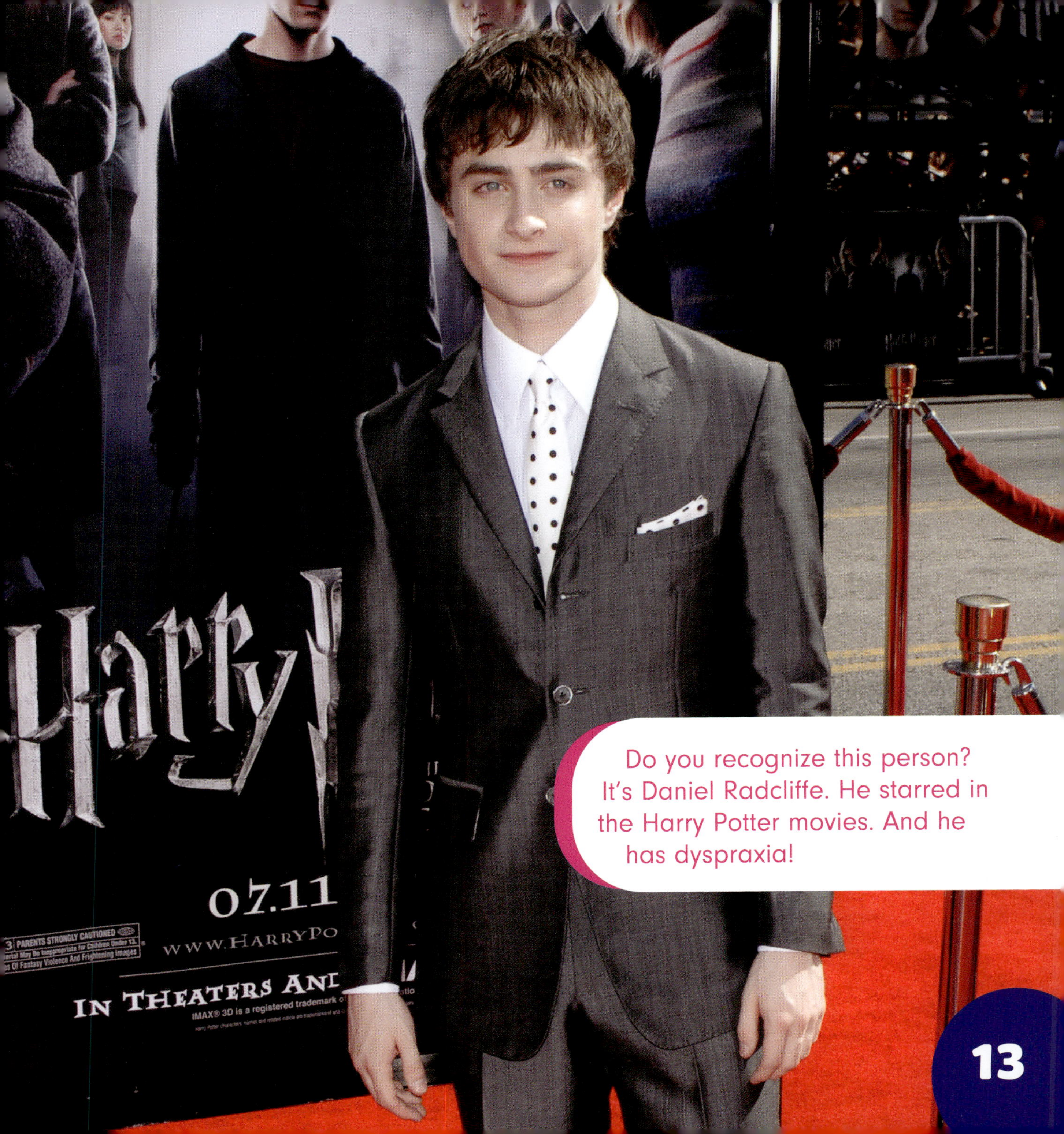

Do you recognize this person? It's Daniel Radcliffe. He starred in the Harry Potter movies. And he has dyspraxia!

ADHD

You may have heard of ADHD. It's a common **disorder**. The letters stand for attention deficit/hyperactivity disorder. Some authorities think it's a learning difference; some don't. But it can certainly affect your ability to learn!

If you have ADHD, you might squirm in your seat and have trouble sitting still. It might be hard to pay attention. You may make **careless** mistakes because it's hard to pay attention to **details**. You may talk a lot, even when it's not your turn. You may forget and lose things a lot. Different people can show ADHD in very different ways.

Your Point of View

Have you heard of Albert Einstein? He's one of the most famous scientists who ever lived. And it's believed he had ADHD!

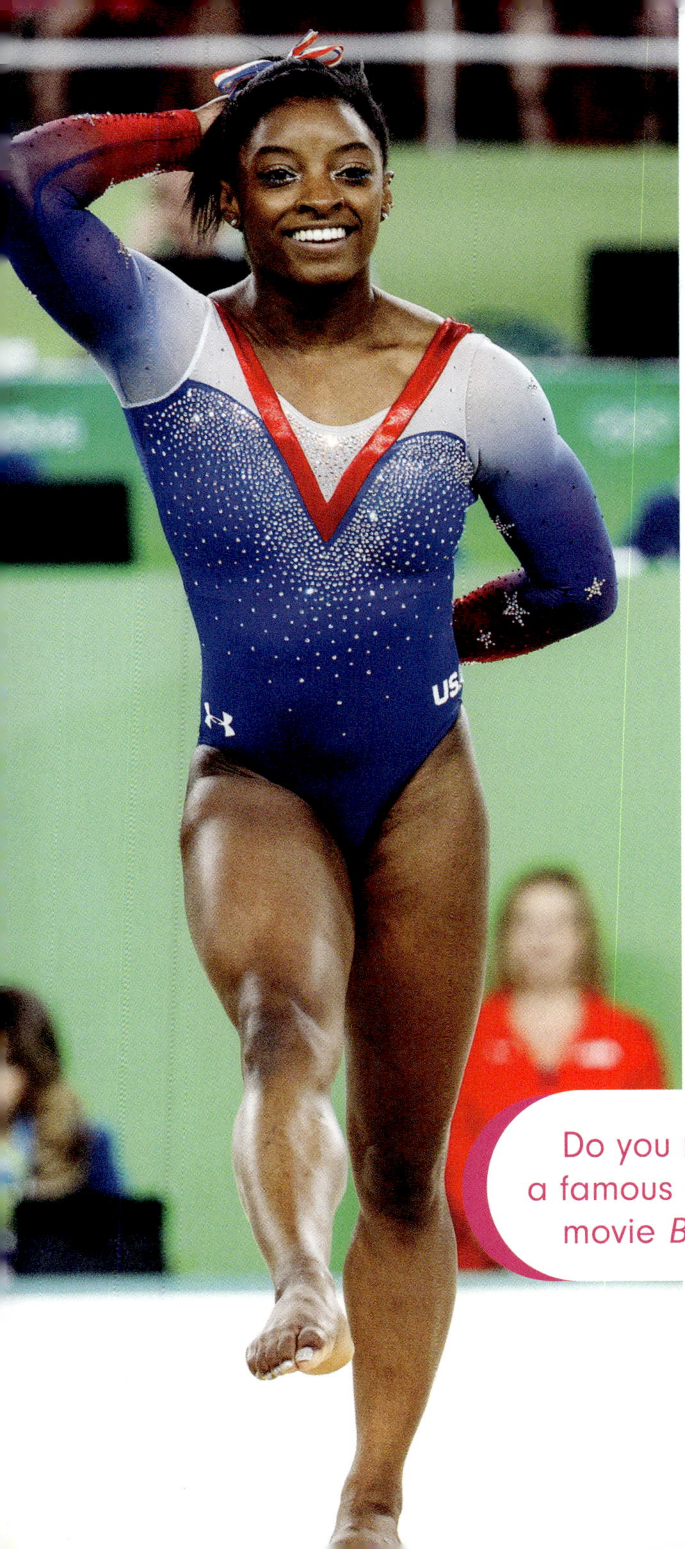

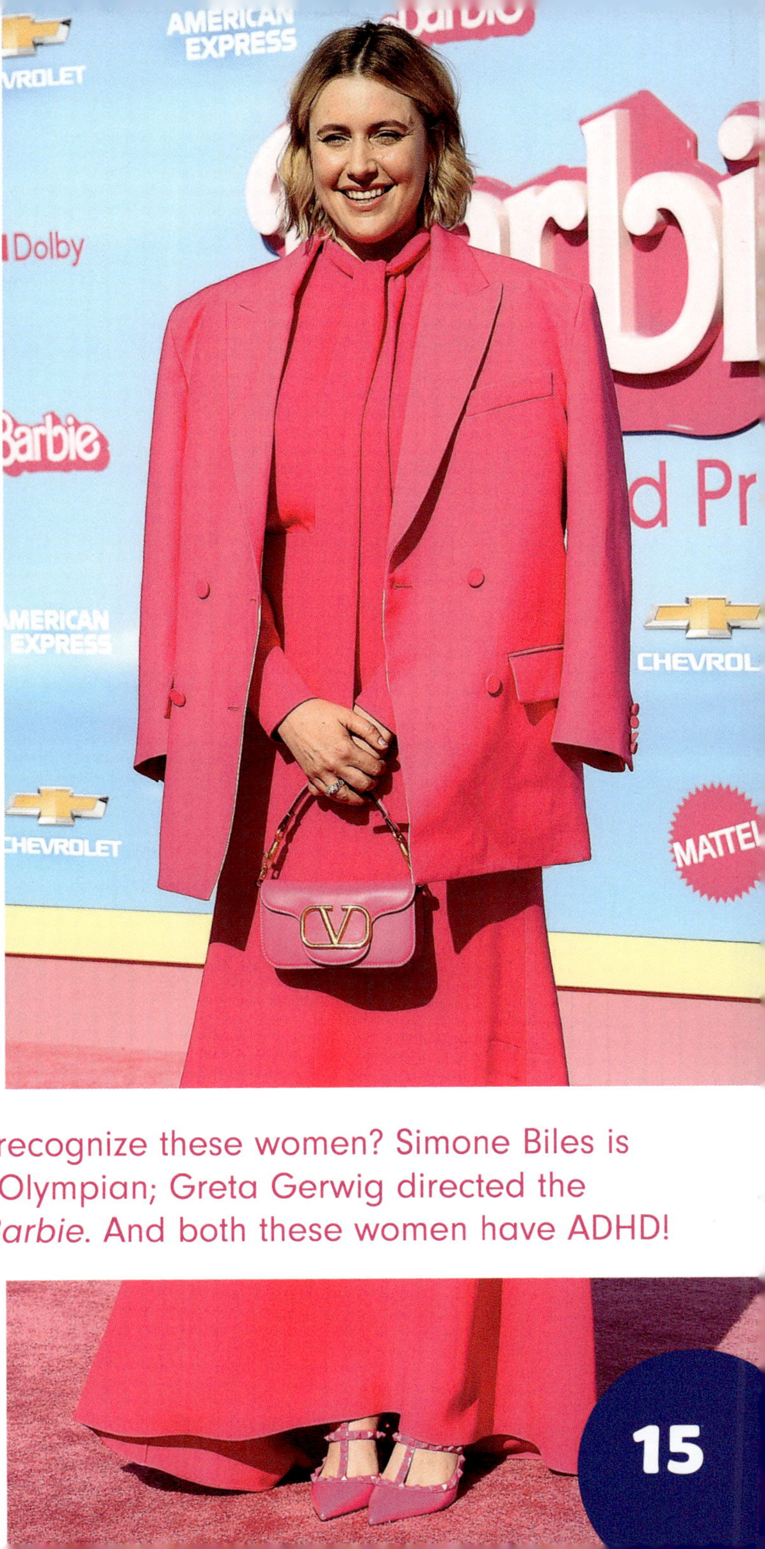

Do you recognize these women? Simone Biles is a famous Olympian; Greta Gerwig directed the movie *Barbie*. And both these women have ADHD!

School Plans

If you have a learning difference, school can be tough sometimes. But laws require schools to help students with learning differences—for free!

Your school may give you a special learning plan called an individual education plan, or IEP. You may also go to special classes. Or you might be covered by something called a 504 plan. That means your school will provide you with **accommodations** such as extra time to complete tasks.

Your Point of View

Two main laws spell out the rights of students with learning differences. One is the Individuals with Disabilities Education Act, which covers IEPs. The other is the Rehabilitation Act, which covers 504 plans.

If you have an IEP, you have a team working to help you. That includes parents or other adults who take care of you, your regular teacher, your special education teacher, and other school officials.

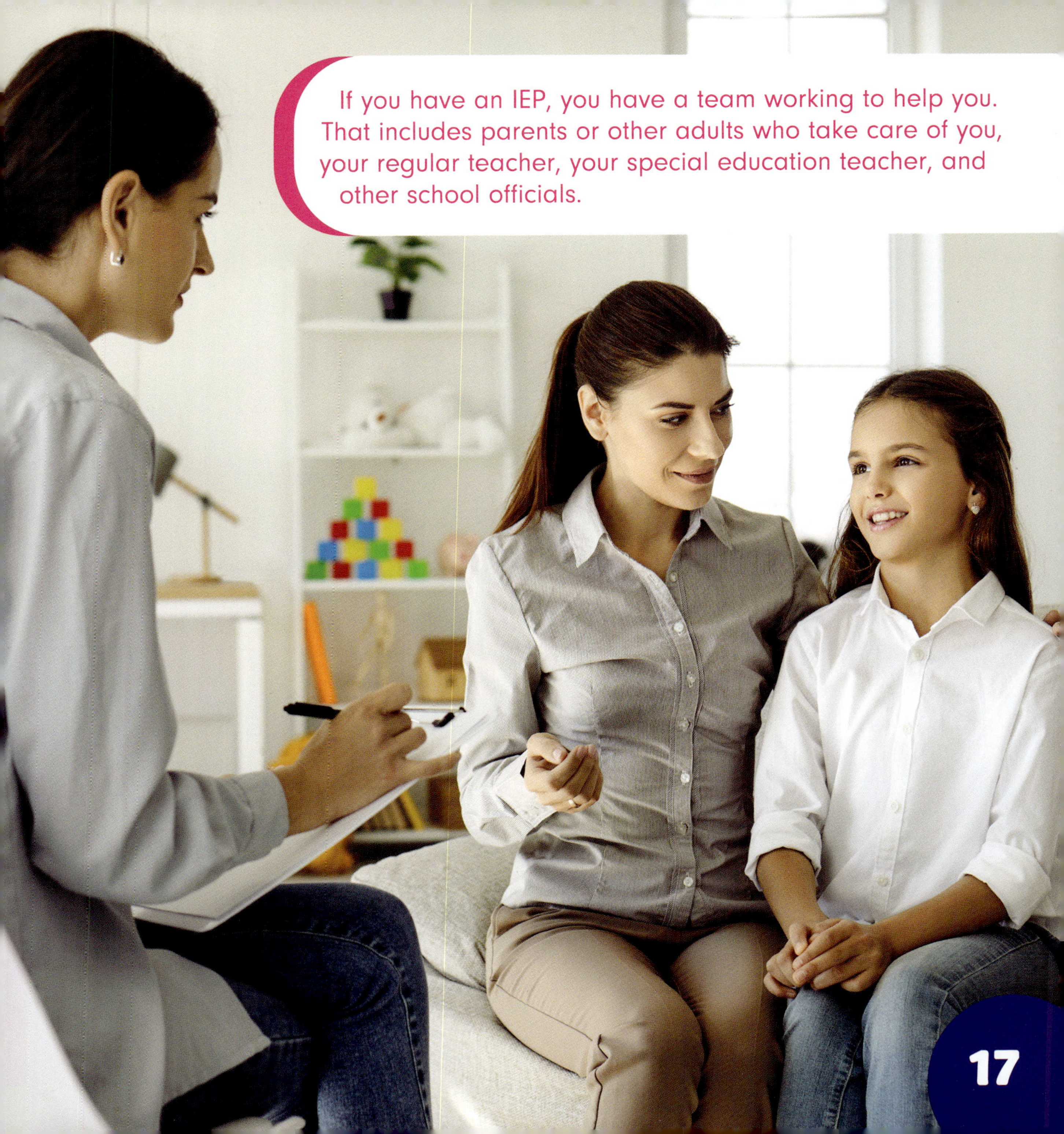

You Can Do It!

Remember, having a learning difference doesn't have anything to do with how smart you are. As you've learned, many successful people have learning differences. And while your school will help you, there are things you can do to help yourself.

If you get upset, place your hands on your stomach and try to grow calm. When you're solving problems, think them through step by step. Record classroom lessons instead of taking notes if it helps you. Remember you have strengths as well as weaknesses. Think about those!

Your Point of View

An authority on dyslexia has said, "Dyslexia is an island of weakness surrounded by a sea of strengths." Whatever learning difference you have, think about it like that—just an island surrounded by a sea of all your strengths!

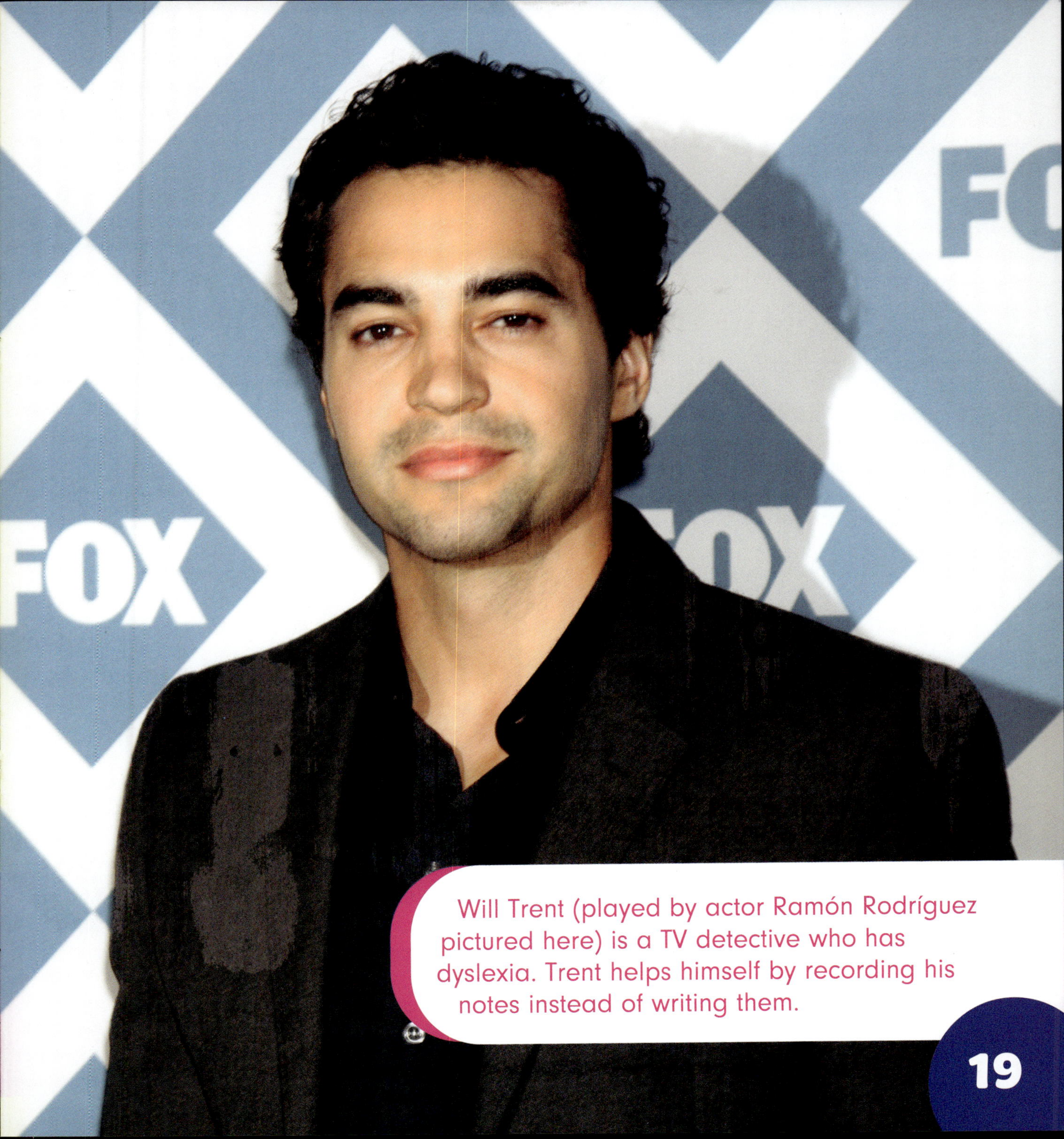

Will Trent (played by actor Ramón Rodríguez pictured here) is a TV detective who has dyslexia. Trent helps himself by recording his notes instead of writing them.

Talk About It

One of the best ways to help yourself is to tell people about your learning difference. This might seem scary at first. But you can practice first with a parent or other trusted adult.

Name your learning difference and explain how it affects you. Maybe it's hard for you to hear your teacher when there's other noise. Or maybe you learn better listening to recorded text than reading it. Tell people! Once others understand what's going on, they can work with you better.

Your Point of View

Maybe it's hard for you to sit still, so you need to take breaks and get up and move around.

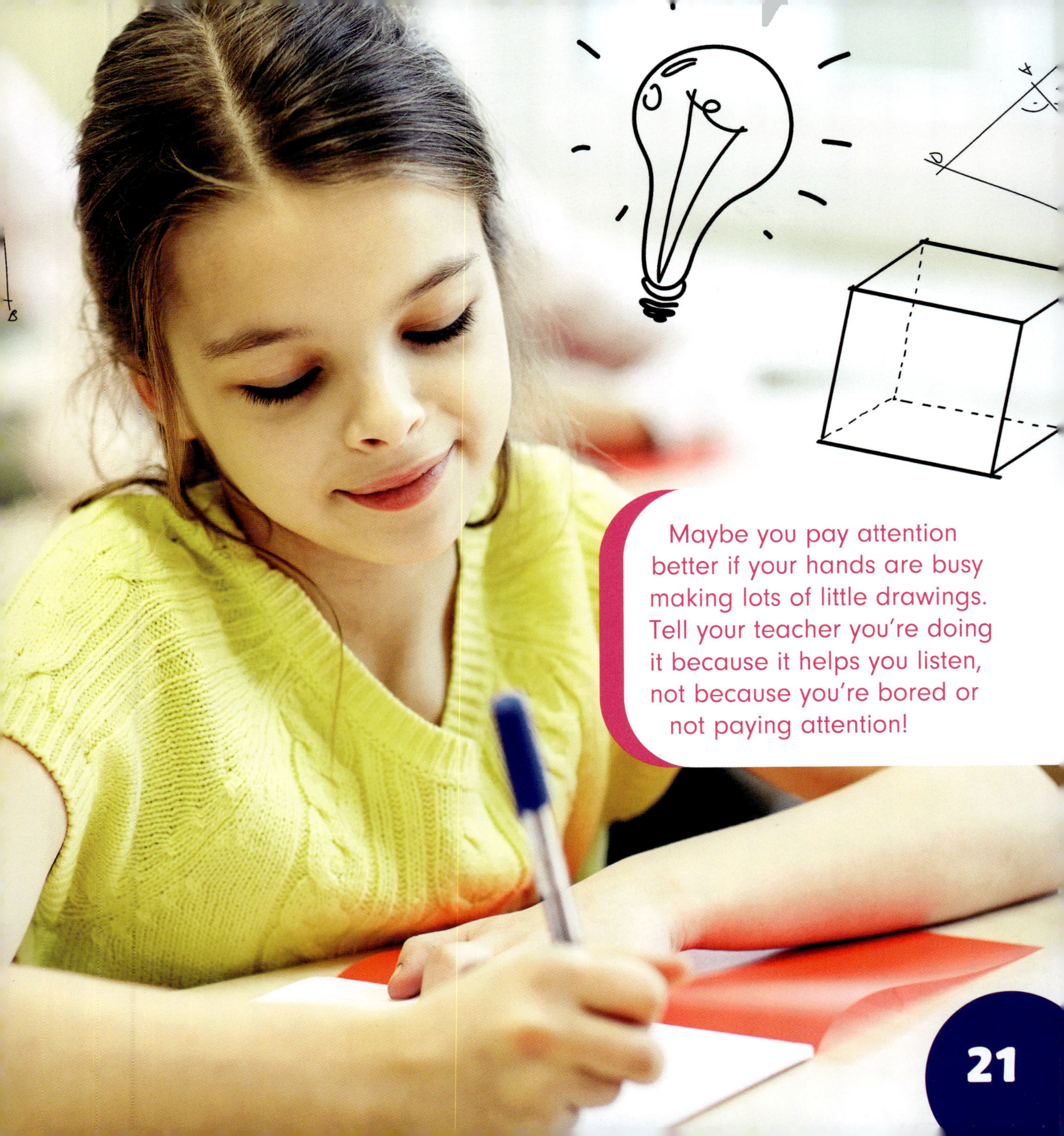

Maybe you pay attention better if your hands are busy making lots of little drawings. Tell your teacher you're doing it because it helps you listen, not because you're bored or not paying attention!

Glossary

accommodation: Something that is done to meet a need.

careless: Not being careful.

coordination: Skillful and balanced body movements.

detail: A small part of something.

disorder: A health condition that is different from the usual.

Founding Father: One of the men who helped create the government of the young United States.

muscle: One of the parts of the body that allow movement.

process: A series of steps or actions taken to complete something.

scissors: A tool made from two blades joined in the middle, with the sharp sides facing each other, that's used for cutting paper and other thin materials.

For More Information

Books

Duhig, Holly. *A Book About ADHD*. New York, NY: PowerKids Press, 2020.

Schuh, Mari. *My Life with Dyslex*ia. North Mankato, MN: The Creative Company, 2021.

Websites

Improving Literacy
improvingliteracy.org/kid-zone/play
Play games and have fun practicing literacy skills!

Kids Health
kidshealth.org/en/kids/adhdkid.html
Learn more about life with ADHD.

Index

A
ADHD, 14, 15

B
Biles, Simone, 15

C
Christie, Agatha, 11

D
dyscalculia, 8, 9
dysgraphia, 10, 11
dyslexia, 6, 7, 18, 19
dyspraxia, 12, 13

E
Einstein, Albert, 14

G
Gerwig, Greta, 15

I
individual education plan (IEP), 16, 17
Individuals with Disabilities Education Act, 16

R
Radcliffe, Daniel, 13
Rehabilitation Act, 16

W
Washington, George, 6